CODY SMITH

300 Squats a Day 30 Day Challenge

Workout Your Glutes, Quadriceps, and Hamstrings While Improving Your Balance and Core Strength With This Lower Body Exercise Program

First published by Nelaco Press 2021

Copyright © 2021 by Cody Smith

First edition

ISBN: 978-1-952381-10-2

This book was professionally typeset on Reedsy.
Find out more at reedsy.com

Contents

Contents

Before You Begin

Hey reader, thanks for grabbing a copy of the book.

If you are looking to pair this workout program with a complimentary guide to shed weight and boost your growth hormones to build more muscle faster, then I've got you covered.

Seems crazy to do both at the same time, but you can.

Better still, it is stupid easy.

Oh, and it is free. You can do this method anytime you want, anywhere for the rest of your life.

I usually sell this information, but I want you to have it.

You can get a copy from your cell phone from a simple text.

Seriously, get your phone out and text BOOST to (678) 506-7543.

Cheers!

Introduction: How to Use This Book

Let me be the first to welcome you to the 300 squats a day 30 day challenge program.

The next 30 days are going to be awesome as you work your way to completing literally 9000 squats.

Squats are an awesome lower body exercise that you can do literally anywhere. Your body is the only gym you need and there are no excuses for skipping leg day.

Since this program is designed to be performed every single day, each workout is not focused on completely obliterating your legs to the point where you can't stand up the next morning.

Each workout is strategically designed to give you the optimum ratio of time your muscles are under tension and time your muscles are under rest so that you can perform it again the next day and not hate yourself.

The beginner workouts have less time under tension per set but take longer to complete the workout. The intermediate and advanced workouts have more time under tension making them significantly harder to perform but you are rewarded with a faster workout.

Before you wonder which workout to start with, I want you to know that there is zero guesswork required of where you need to start.

This program starts with an initial squat assessment to determine where you need to start in the program. Don't skip the assessment.

Once you complete the assessment, your 30 day challenge will start the very next day with whatever workout you're assigned from the post-assessment results.

While you're starting out in the program, you'll most likely be very sore early on in the program. Your body has not adapted to completing 300 squats a day yet. That's okay, if the soreness is bearable, you can continue with the program.

If the soreness is unbearable, take a break for a few days until you recover and hop right back into the program where you left off.

If you can't complete your workout one day or have to skip a day here and there, don't fret. That's 300% okay and won't throw you way off. Quitting is the only failure.

Remember, this is a challenge. It's supposed to be challenging.

If it's too easy, the only thing you've gained is wasted time.

This brings me to the most important question:

Are you ready to accept the challenge?

With that said, welcome to the 300 squats a day challenge.

Head to the initial squat assessment and let the games begin.

Initial Squat Assessment

Welcome to the initial squat assessment portion of this program. This is where we're going to check your current repetition count to see how many squats you can actually perform without stopping.

This number will determine which workout you need to start with as you make your way through the 300 squat challenge program.

Make sure you are doing full squats going all the way through the motion. Proper form is key to getting the most out of this exercise so I'll quickly go over how to properly perform a squat.

You're going to start the exercise by standing with your feet shoulder-width apart with your toes pointed slightly outward. Begin the squat by squatting back as if you are going to sit in a chair keeping all or most of your weight on your heels so you don't lean forward. You have completed the descend when your upper thighs are parallel to the floor. Ascend back up to the starting position. The is one rep.

Throughout the motion, your back should not bend.

Go ahead complete as many squats as you can without stopping.

When you're done, make a note of how many you completed and head to the post assessment results section.

Post Assessment Results

Welcome to the post assessment results section.

This is where you'll see what workout you'll start with based on the number of squats you completed during the assessment.

Still got that number in your head?

Good.

- If you completed <18 squats, your first workout starting tomorrow will be Workout 1.
- If you completed between 18 - 24 squats, your first workout will be Workout 2.
- If you completed between 25 - 29 squats, your first workout will be Workout 3.
- If you completed between 30 - 32 squats, your first workout will be Workout 4.
- If you completed between 33 - 38 squats, your first workout will be Workout 5.
- If you completed between 39 - 44 squats, your first workout will be Workout 6.
- If you completed between 45 - 47squats, your first workout will be

Workout 7.

- If you completed between 48 - 53 squats, your first workout will be Workout 8.
- If you completed between 54 - 59 squats, your first workout will be Workout 9.
- If you completed between 60 - 62 squats, your first workout will be Workout 10.
- If you completed between 63 - 68 squats, your first workout will be Workout 11.
- If you completed between 69 - 74 squats, your first workout will be Workout 12.
- If you completed between 75 - 77 squats, your first workout will be Workout 13.
- If you completed between 78 - 83 squats, your first workout will be Workout 14.
- If you completed between 84 - 89 squats, your first workout will be Workout 15.
- If you completed 90 or more squats, your first workout will be Workout 16.

Don't fret if you didn't complete a lot of squats. The point of the challenge is to start where you are and complete the full 30 days of 300 squats a day. Not to be some amazing squat champion on day 1.

With that said, you know where you need to start starting tomorrow with your very first 300 squats a day workout.

See you there.

Completed Workouts Checklist

Check these off as you complete them:

_____Workout 1

_____Workout 2

_____Workout 3

_____Workout 4

_____Workout 5

_____Workout 6

_____Workout 7

_____Workout 8

_____Workout 9

_____Workout 10

_____Workout 11

_____Workout 12

_____Workout 13

_____Workout 14

_____Workout 15

_____Workout 16

30 Day Completion Checklist

Date started: _____ (DD/MM/YYYY)

_____Day 1

_____Day 2

_____Day 3

_____Day 4

_____Day 5

_____Day 6

_____Day 7

_____Day 8

_____Day 9

_____Day 10

_____Day 11

_____Day 12

_____Day 13

_____Day 14

_____Day 15

_____Day 16

_____Day 17

_____Day 18

_____Day 19

_____Day 20

_____Day 21

_____Day 22

_____Day 23

_____Day 24
_____Day 25
_____Day 26
_____Day 27
_____Day 28
_____Day 29
_____Day 30

Pre and Post Challenge Measurements

The following measurements are 100% optional and are not required to start or finish the program. I know some people will be curious to know other areas that are positively affected by completing the challenge.

Starting weight: _____

Starting squat rep max: _____

Starting squat max: _____

Starting deadlift max: _____

Starting leg press max: _____

Starting right thigh measurement: _____

Ending weight: _____

Ending squat rep max: _____

Ending squat max: _____

Ending deadlift max: _____

Ending leg press max: _____

Ending right thigh measurement: _____

Workout 1

Welcome to Workout 1 of the 300 squats a day 30 day challenge.

For this workout, 3 squats is performed every minute.

Because this is such a long workout, do your best to at least complete 50 squats. Once you get stronger, re-do the initial assessment to work your way up the workout chain where the workouts are harder but take less time to complete.

This workout is way easier with an interval timer app. I suggest downloading one onto your phone with the following settings for this workout:

Intervals: 100

Time per interval: 1:06

That time will give you enough time to complete the number of correct squats and enough time to rest between sets. The interval app also makes it easy to determine what set you're on.

With that said, go ahead and get started.

Come back in when you are done.

* * *

Way to go!

You completed 300 squats today!

If that workout was too easy, consider moving up to the next workout.

If that workout was still fairly challenging, continue with this workout tomorrow.

That's all I've got for you today. See you tomorrow, champ!

Workout 2

Welcome to Workout 2 of the 300 squats a day 30 day challenge.

For this workout, 3 or 6 squats are performed every minute.

The first 25 sets are 6 squats each.

The last 50 sets are 3 squat each.

Because this is such a long workout, do your best to at least complete 50 squats. Once you get stronger, re-do the initial assessment to work your way up the workout chain where the workouts are harder but take less time to complete.

This workout is way easier with an interval timer app. I suggest downloading one onto your phone with the following settings for this workout:

Intervals: 75

Time per interval: 1:12

That time will give you enough time to complete the number of correct squats and enough time to rest between sets. The interval app also makes it easy to determine what set you're on.

With that said, go ahead and get started.

Come back in when you are done.

* * *

Way to go!

You completed 300 squats today!

If that workout was too easy, consider moving up to the next workout.

If that workout was still fairly challenging, continue with this workout tomorrow.

That's all I've got for you today. See you tomorrow, champ!

Workout 3

Welcome to Workout 3 of the 300 squats a day 30 day challenge.

For this workout, 3 or 6 squats are performed every minute.

The first 40 sets are 6 squats each.

The last 20 sets are 3 squat each.

Because this is such a long workout, do your best to at least complete 50 squats. Once you get stronger, re-do the initial assessment to work your way up the workout chain where the workouts are harder but take less time to complete.

This workout is way easier with an interval timer app. I suggest downloading one onto your phone with the following settings for this workout:

Intervals: 60

Time per interval: 1:12

That time will give you enough time to complete the number of correct squats and enough time to rest between sets. The interval app also makes it easy to determine what set you're on.

With that said, go ahead and get started.

Come back in when you are done.

* * *

Way to go!

You completed 300 squats today!

If that workout was too easy, consider moving up to the next workout.

If that workout was still fairly challenging, continue with this workout tomorrow.

That's all I've got for you today. See you tomorrow, champ!

Workout 4

Welcome to Workout 1 of the 300 squats a day 30 day challenge.

For this workout, 6 squats are performed every minute.

Because this is such a long workout, do your best to at least complete 50 squats. Once you get stronger, re-do the initial assessment to work your way up the workout chain where the workouts are harder but take less time to complete.

This workout is way easier with an interval timer app. I suggest downloading one onto your phone with the following settings for this workout:

Intervals: 50

Time per interval: 1:12

That time will give you enough time to complete the number of correct squats and enough time to rest between sets. The interval app also makes it easy to determine what set you're on.

With that said, go ahead and get started.

Come back in when you are done.

* * *

Way to go!

You completed 300 squats today!

If that workout was too easy, consider moving up to the next workout.

If that workout was still fairly challenging, continue with this workout tomorrow.

That's all I've got for you today. See you tomorrow, champ!

Workout 5

Welcome to Workout 5 of the 300 squats a day 30 day challenge.

For this workout, 6 or 9 squats are performed every minute.

The first 14 sets are 9 squats each.

The last 29 sets are 6 squats each.

This workout is way easier with an interval timer app. I suggest downloading one onto your phone with the following settings for this workout:

Intervals: 43

Time per interval: 1:18

That time will give you enough time to complete the number of correct squats and enough time to rest between sets. The interval app also makes it easy to determine what set you're on.

With that said, go ahead and get started.

Come back in when you are done.

* * *

Way to go!

You completed 300 squats today!

If that workout was too easy, consider moving up to the next workout.

If that workout was still fairly challenging, continue with this workout tomorrow.

That's all I've got for you today. See you tomorrow, champ!

Workout 6

Welcome to Workout 6 of the 300 squats a day 30 day challenge.

For this workout, 6 or 9 squats are performed every minute.

The first 24 sets are 9 squats each.

The last 14 sets are 6 squats each.

This workout is way easier with an interval timer app. I suggest downloading one onto your phone with the following settings for this workout:

Intervals: 38

Time per interval: 1:18

That time will give you enough time to complete the number of correct squats and enough time to rest between sets. The interval app also makes it easy to determine what set you're on.

With that said, go ahead and get started.

Come back in when you are done.

* * *

Way to go!

You completed 300 squats today!

If that workout was too easy, consider moving up to the next workout.

If that workout was still fairly challenging, continue with this workout tomorrow.

That's all I've got for you today. See you tomorrow, champ!

Workout 7

Welcome to Workout 7 of the 300 squats a day 30 day challenge.

For this workout, 9 squats are performed every minute.

The first 33 sets are 9 squats each.

The last set is 3 squats.

This workout is way easier with an interval timer app. I suggest downloading one onto your phone with the following settings for this workout:

Intervals: 34

Time per interval: 1:18

That time will give you enough time to complete the number of correct squats and enough time to rest between sets. The interval app also makes it easy to determine what set you're on.

With that said, go ahead and get started.

Come back in when you are done.

* * *

Way to go!

You completed 300 squats today!

If that workout was too easy, consider moving up to the next workout.

If that workout was still fairly challenging, continue with this workout tomorrow.

That's all I've got for you today. See you tomorrow, champ!

Workout 8

Welcome to Workout 8 of the 300 squats a day 30 day challenge.

For this workout, 9 or 12 squats are performed every minute.

The first 10 sets are 12 squats each.

The last 20 sets are 9 squats each.

This workout is way easier with an interval timer app. I suggest downloading one onto your phone with the following settings for this workout:

Intervals: 30

Time per interval: 1:24

That time will give you enough time to complete the number of correct squats and enough time to rest between sets. The interval app also makes it easy to determine what set you're on.

With that said, go ahead and get started.

Come back in when you are done.

* * *

Way to go!

You completed 300 squats today!

If that workout was too easy, consider moving up to the next workout.

If that workout was still fairly challenging, continue with this workout tomorrow.

That's all I've got for you today. See you tomorrow, champ!

Workout 9

Welcome to Workout 9 of the 300 squats a day 30 day challenge.

For this workout, 9 or 12 squats are performed every minute.

The first 18 sets are 12 squats each.

The next 9 sets are 9 squats each.

The last set is 3 squats.

This workout is way easier with an interval timer app. I suggest downloading one onto your phone with the following settings for this workout:

Intervals: 28

Time per interval: 1:24

That time will give you enough time to complete the number of correct squats and enough time to rest between sets. The interval app also makes it easy to determine what set you're on.

With that said, go ahead and get started.

Come back in when you are done.

* * *

Way to go!

You completed 300 squats today!

If that workout was too easy, consider moving up to the next workout.

If that workout was still fairly challenging, continue with this workout tomorrow.

That's all I've got for you today. See you tomorrow, champ!

Workout 10

Welcome to Workout 10 of the 300 squats a day 30 day challenge.

For this workout, 12 squats are performed every minute.

This workout is way easier with an interval timer app. I suggest downloading one onto your phone with the following settings for this workout:

Intervals: 25

Time per interval: 1:24

That time will give you enough time to complete the number of correct squats and enough time to rest between sets. The interval app also makes it easy to determine what set you're on.

With that said, go ahead and get started.

Come back in when you are done.

* * *

Way to go!

You completed 300 squats today!

If that workout was too easy, consider moving up to the next workout.

If that workout was still fairly challenging, continue with this workout tomorrow.

That's all I've got for you today. See you tomorrow, champ!

Workout 11

Welcome to Workout 11 of the 300 squats a day 30 day challenge.

For this workout, 12 or 15 squats are performed every minute.

The first 8 sets are 15 squats each.

The last 15 sets are 12 squats each.

This workout is way easier with an interval timer app. I suggest downloading one onto your phone with the following settings for this workout:

Intervals: 23

Time per interval: 1:30

That time will give you enough time to complete the number of correct squats and enough time to rest between sets. The interval app also makes it easy to determine what set you're on.

With that said, go ahead and get started.

Come back in when you are done.

* * *

Way to go!

You completed 300 squats today!

If that workout was too easy, consider moving up to the next workout.

If that workout was still fairly challenging, continue with this workout tomorrow.

That's all I've got for you today. See you tomorrow, champ!

Workout 12

Welcome to Workout 12 of the 300 squats a day 30 day challenge.

For this workout, 12 or 15 squats are performed every minute.

The first 14 sets are 15 squats each.

The next 7 sets are 12 squats each.

The last set is 6 squats.

This workout is way easier with an interval timer app. I suggest downloading one onto your phone with the following settings for this workout:

Intervals: 22

Time per interval: 1:30

That time will give you enough time to complete the number of correct squats and enough time to rest between sets. The interval app also makes it easy to determine what set you're on.

With that said, go ahead and get started.

Come back in when you are done.

* * *

Way to go!

You completed 300 squats today!

If that workout was too easy, consider moving up to the next workout.

If that workout was still fairly challenging, continue with this workout tomorrow.

That's all I've got for you today. See you tomorrow, champ!

Workout 13

Welcome to Workout 13 of the 300 squats a day 30 day challenge.

For this workout, 15 squats are performed every minute.

This workout is way easier with an interval timer app. I suggest downloading one onto your phone with the following settings for this workout:

Intervals: 20

Time per interval: 1:30

That time will give you enough time to complete the number of correct squats and enough time to rest between sets. The interval app also makes it easy to determine what set you're on.

With that said, go ahead and get started.

Come back in when you are done.

* * *

Way to go!

You completed 300 squats today!

If that workout was too easy, consider moving up to the next workout.

If that workout was still fairly challenging, continue with this workout tomorrow.

That's all I've got for you today. See you tomorrow, champ!

Workout 14

Welcome to Workout 14 of the 300 squats a day 30 day challenge.

For this workout, 15 or 18 squats are performed every minute.

The first 6 sets are 18 squats each.

The next 12 sets are 15 squats each.

The last set is 12 squats.

This workout is way easier with an interval timer app. I suggest downloading one onto your phone with the following settings for this workout:

Intervals: 19

Time per interval: 1:36

That time will give you enough time to complete the number of correct squats and enough time to rest between sets. The interval app also makes it easy to determine what set you're on.

With that said, go ahead and get started.

Come back in when you are done.

* * *

Way to go!

You completed 300 squats today!

If that workout was too easy, consider moving up to the next workout.

If that workout was still fairly challenging, continue with this workout tomorrow.

That's all I've got for you today. See you tomorrow, champ!

Workout 15

Welcome to Workout 15 of the 300 squats a day 30 day challenge.

For this workout, 15 or 18 squats are performed every minute.

The first 11 sets are 18 squats each.

The next 6 sets are 15 squats each.

The last set is 12 squats.

This workout is way easier with an interval timer app. I suggest downloading one onto your phone with the following settings for this workout:

Intervals: 18

Time per interval: 1:36

That time will give you enough time to complete the number of correct squats and enough time to rest between sets. The interval app also makes it easy to determine what set you're on.

With that said, go ahead and get started.

Come back in when you are done.

* * *

Way to go!

You completed 300 squats today!

If that workout was too easy, consider moving up to the next workout.

If that workout was still fairly challenging, continue with this workout tomorrow.

That's all I've got for you today. See you tomorrow, champ!

Workout 16

Welcome to Workout 16 of the 300 squats a day 30 day challenge.

For this workout, 18 squats are performed every minute.

The first 16 sets are 18 squats each.

The last set is 12 squats.

This workout is way easier with an interval timer app. I suggest downloading one onto your phone with the following settings for this workout:

Intervals: 17

Time per interval: 1:36

That time will give you enough time to complete the number of correct squats and enough time to rest between sets. The interval app also makes it easy to determine what set you're on.

With that said, go ahead and get started.

Come back in when you are done.

* * *

Way to go!

You completed 300 squats today!

That's more than most people do in a year.

That's all I've got for you today. See you tomorrow, champ!

Post 30 Day Assessment

Hey champ, before we get into the post-assessment, I'd like to ask you for a quick favor.

I'm going to be greedy for a minute here and ask you to leave a review for the book.

Maybe give a star for every time your legs shook right after completing a workout.

Reviews are a pain to get but it'll only take a minute or two to leave one.

So while you're warming up to destroy this assessment, pull your phone out and scan this QR code.

It'll take you straight to the book's page on Amazon.

Scroll to the bottom and click 'Leave a Customer Review.' Leave a star rating, say a few words, and click submit.

It's that simple!

Once you're done, come back to crush your assessment.

* * *

You accepted the 30 day challenge, you completed the 30 day challenge, and now it's time to see where you are now after nailing down 9000 squats.

This is pretty exciting.

All that hard work, dedication, and blisters to get to this point.

I hope to goodness' sake you've allowed a couple of days to recover between the 30th day of your challenge and now.

You'll see much better results that way.

With that said, get ready to crush this assessment.

Remember that number you started out with during the first assessment?

Go ahead and say that number out loud.

You're about to blow past that number.

Go ahead complete as many squats as you can without stopping.

* * *

How'd you do?

Satisfied with your new number?

Yes and no right?

Yes because you knocked out way more reps and no because you're hungry for more!

Don't be afraid to take a week off and start the challenge again with your new assessment number.

Conclusion

Hey champ, I really hope you enjoyed the 300 squats a day 30 day program.

I hope it was challenging, I hope you pushed yourself, and I hope your post-assessment was worthy of a killer high five.

If you're thirsty for more challenges, we've got more where this came from.

And if you've enjoyed this book, do take a second to leave a review.

Those jokers are hard to get but will only take a minute or two for you to leave one.

Until next time, champ.

Conclusion

Made in the USA
Monee, IL
09 August 2024

63559012R00038